YOUR KNOWLEDGE HAS VALUE

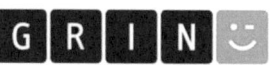

Bibliographic information published by the German National Library:

The German National Library lists this publication in the National Bibliography; detailed bibliographic data are available on the Internet at http://dnb.dnb.de .

Imprint:

Copyright © 2018 GRIN Verlag
Print and binding: Books on Demand GmbH, Norderstedt Germany
ISBN: 9783668627857

This book at GRIN:

https://www.grin.com/document/388763

Patrick Kimuyu

Understanding Schizophrenia

GRIN Verlag

GRIN - Your knowledge has value

Since its foundation in 1998, GRIN has specialized in publishing academic texts by students, college teachers and other academics as e-book and printed book. The website www.grin.com is an ideal platform for presenting term papers, final papers, scientific essays, dissertations and specialist books.

Visit us on the internet:

http://www.grin.com/

http://www.facebook.com/grincom

http://www.twitter.com/grin_com

Understanding Schizophrenia

Patrick Kimuyu

Abstract

Schizophrenia is a psychotic disorder affecting all people, worldwide. Its prevalence is higher among males than females in which its onset is 25 years and 27 years in men and women, respectively.

The causes of this disorder are associated with genetic and environmental factors. Some genetic factors increase vulnerability of an individual to the disease, whereas environmental factors trigger the disease in vulnerable individuals.

Its main signs and symptoms include delusions, disorganized speech, catatonic behavior, and hallucinations.

Diagnosis of schizophrenia is based on DSM and ICD-10 criteria, and it involves differential diagnosis of other psychotic and medical issues.

Overall, the pathophysiology of this illness is related to abnormalities in brain structure, neurotransmitter and immune system. As such, treatment aims at addressing the symptoms of the disorder in which antipsychotic medication and psychosocial interventions serve as the main treatment approaches.

Regarding prognosis of schizophrenia, inadequate access to healthcare increases mortality. Suicide is one of the main causes of mortality among people with schizophrenia.

Conclusively, schizophrenia presents immense challenges, but research has been instrumental in improving its diagnosis and treatment.

Introduction

Schizophrenia is a psychotic disorder that presents immense challenges to psychiatrists, as well as, other public health personnel. The complexity of this disorder is attributable to its debilitating effects. It affects an individual's social functioning, behavior and thoughts, thus making it difficult for social interactions. Epidemiological data indicate that 0.3 to 0.7% of the global population is affected by Schizophrenia (Van Os & Kapur, 2009). However, its prevalence exhibits demographic inequalities in which the disorder occurs 1.4 times among males compared to females (Picchioni & Murray, 2007). Similarly, its onset occurs at different peak ages. This condition is report to occur early in men with the peak age of onset being 25 years compared to females whose peak age of onset is 27 years (Cascio, Cella, Preti, Meneghelli & Cocchi, 2012). According to Kumra, Shaw, Merka, Nakayama & Augustin (2001), onset of schizophrenia is rare during childhood. Overall, schizophrenia exhibits similar trends in incidence and prevalence, worldwide. On the other hand, schizophrenia causes many deaths and it is also responsible for 1% of disability adjusted life years (Picchioni & Murray, 2007). For instance, 20,000 schizophrenia-related deaths occurred in 2010 (Lozano, Naghavi & Foreman, 2012). Concisely, schizophrenia has immense clinical and psychosocial implications. This is why this term paper is intended to provide a comprehensive overview of schizophrenia.

Causes of Schizophrenia

From a critical analysis, the causes of schizophrenia remain unclear. However, it is apparent that the onset of the disorder is related to a mystic interplay between environmental and genetic factors. Over the decades, schizophrenia has been found to exhibit hereditary traits. This implies that hereditary factors are involved in the occurrence of the disorder. The hereditary component of schizophrenia is evidenced by genetic studies in which first-degree relatives have been found to develop the disorder more than the general population. It is reported that the risk of developing schizophrenia is 1% and 10% in general population and first-degree relatives, respectively. However, it is worth noting that genetic predisposition only influences schizophrenia's onset, because there are not hereditary genes that links genetics with the cause of the disorder. These revelations are based on actual epidemiological data that shows that 60% of people with schizophrenia do not a family history of the disorder.

On the other hand, environmental factors are believed to have an immense impact on the onset of schizophrenia. Clinical studies reveal that environmental factors triggers schizophrenia in vulnerable individuals, especially those who possess inherited genetic

2

components that increase the disorder's vulnerability. This phenomenon has been confirmed by twin and adoption studies, and extensive research on the same is ongoing, in order to unravel the underlying pathological factors. Another significant environmental factor that has been found to cause schizophrenia is psychosocial stress. Ordinarily, stress and anxiety have been found to impair cognitive functioning. In this context, increases in cortisol levels which are caused by stress are believed to trigger schizophrenia. Similarly, other stress-inducing environmental factors have been linked with the development of schizophrenia. Some of these factors include exposure to viral infections, especially during prenatal or infancy, childhood sexual or physical abuse, and oxygen insufficiency during birth. Family issues such as early parental separation or death have also been found to play key roles in the development of schizophrenia among adults.

Abnormalities in brain structure and chemistry have also been associated with the development of schizophrenia. The fact that schizophrenia affects cognition implies that the respective brain regions are affected. For instance, the enlargement of brain ventricles among most schizophrenics reveals that abnormalities in the volume of brain tissue are linked to schizophrenia (Wright, Rabe-Hesketh & Woodruff, 2000). Another correlation is obtained from the abnormalities in the frontal lobe. Most schizophrenics exhibit low activity in this lobe which is responsible for decision-making, reasoning and planning. Moreover, abnormalities in amygdale, hippocampus and temporal lobes have been associated with the development of schizophrenia.

Signs and Symptoms of Schizophrenia

Ordinarily, the onset of schizophrenia occurs gradually through different phases. It begins with early warning signs before the occurrence of the initial severe episode. However, some individuals experience an abrupt appearance of the disorder without warning signs.

Early Warning Signs

During the early warning phase, most people are observed to exhibit behavioral changes. In most cases, they seem emotionless, unmotivated, eccentric, and reclusive. Some of the most common early signs of this disorder are social withdrawal, hostility, depression, expressionless gaze, forgetfulness, extreme reaction, especially to criticism, and problems in personal hygiene.

On the other hand, full-blown schizophrenia is characterized by five main types of symptoms: delusions, disorganized speech, negative symptoms, disorganized behavior, and hallucinations.

Delusions:

Delusions are the most common occurring symptoms of schizophrenia with over 90% of schizophrenics showing delusions. However, the natures of delusions are diverse although they reflect bizarre or illogical ideas. For instance, some people experience delusions of persecution, whereas others experience delusions of reference, grandeur or control.

Hallucinations:

Hallucinations are strange sounds or sensations in one's mind that are not real. In theory, hallucinations involve the five principal senses, although auditory and visual hallucinations are common among schizophrenics. It has been found out that hallucinations often occur when the person is solitude or alone. In most cases, auditory hallucinations involve voices or sounds that are abusive, vulgar or critical, and this can explain the aggressiveness among schizophrenics.

Disorganized Behavior:

Schizophrenics are observed to show a high degree of cognitive impairment. This is demonstrated by the disruption of goal-oriented activities such as work, social interactions and personal hygiene. In most cases, disorganized behavior is shown by lack of impulse or inhibition control, bizarre behaviors, unpredictable emotional responses, and decline in daily functioning.

Disorganized Speech:

Disorganized speech is another main characteristic of schizophrenia. Ordinarily, schizophrenics experience fragmented thinking which is shown by difficulties in maintaining a line of thought or adequate attention span. The key speech disorganization signs include loose associations between thoughts, neologism, perseveration, and clanging.

Negative Symptoms:

Schizophrenics express the absence of normal behaviors that are expressed by resilient individuals. Some of the most common negative symptoms associated with schizophrenia include social withdrawal, lack of enthusiasm, speech difficulties or absence of emotional expression including restricted facial expression, blank staring and flat voice.

Diagnosis of Schizophrenia

Diagnosis of schizophrenia exhibits difficulties due to its close resemblance to other psychotic disorders. In practice, diagnosis of schizophrenia is based on several aspects. Foremost, a comprehensive psychiatric evaluation and physical examination are essential in effective diagnosis of the disorder. In addition, medical history and clinical laboratory tests aid in the diagnosis of schizophrenia. Psychiatric evaluation involves an inquiry on the psychiatric history, individual's symptoms, and history of mental health problems. On the other hand, medical history and physical examination focus on identifying any underlying medical issues that may be linked to the disorder. Finally, laboratory tests aim at identifying abnormalities in brain structure and chemical balance. It also plays a key role in differential diagnosis to rule out other medical conditions that express similar symptoms with schizophrenia (Lehman, Lieberman, Dixon, McGlashan, Miller, Perkins & Kreyenbuhl, 2010).

In order to ensure accurate diagnosis, comprehensive diagnostic criteria have been developed. Diagnosis can be based, either on the DSM-5 (Diagnostic and Statistical Manual of Mental Disorders) criteria developed by the American Psychiatric Association or the WHO's ICD-10 (International Statistical Classification of Diseases and Related Health Problems) criteria. In the United States, DSM-5 criteria has gained widespread acceptance by psychiatrists. These criteria aim at determining certain severity for diagnosis (Picchioni & Murray, 2007).

Overall, diagnosis is made if two or more of the main symptoms are present for at least 30 days. These symptoms include delusions, negative symptoms, disorganized speech, hallucinations, and catatonic or disorganized behavior. Other key symptoms that should be present include functioning problems such as poor personal hygiene, impaired social interactions and working or schooling problems. In addition, history of continuous occurrence of schizophrenia signs for at least 6 months with the active symptoms persisting for at least 1 month is used in these criteria. Finally, there should be no other medical condition and psychotic disorder diagnosed or substance abuse problem (American Psychiatric Association, 2000).

Conditions with Similar Symptoms with Schizophrenia

In practice, it is recommended that other medical and psychological conditions are ruled out before schizophrenia diagnosis, in order to avoid misdiagnosis. Some of these conditions include other mental health disorders, substance abuse, mood disorders, and Post-traumatic stress disorder (PTSD).

Psychotic Disorders:

There are several psychotic disorders that mimic schizophrenia symptoms. Some of these disorders include brief psychotic disorder, schizophreniform and schizoaffective disorder. Due to the complexity involved in differentiating these disorders from schizophrenia, correct diagnosis may be achieved after more than 6 months.

Substance Abuse:

Addictive substances are known to trigger psychotic symptoms. For instance, drugs such as heroin, cocaine, alcohol, and amphetamines are associated with psychotic symptoms. On the other hand, some prescription and over-the-counter drugs are known to cause psychotic reactions. Therefore, toxicology screening aids in diagnosis substance abuse.

Mood Disorders and PTSD

Mood disorders are believed to mimic schizophrenia, especially mania and depression. In most cases, diagnosis of schizophrenia is complicated by bipolar disorder and depressive disorder because they show similar positive and negative symptoms. For instance, bipolar disorder is characterized by disorganized speech, hallucination and delusions, the main symptoms of schizophrenia. On the other hand, depressive disorder shows social withdrawal, apathy and reduced activity as the key symptoms. These features are considered as negative symptoms for schizophrenic episodes.

Pathophysiology of Schizophrenia

From a clinical perspective, schizophrenia progresses through a particular pathophysiological course. Overall, clinical studies indicate that the pathophysiology is associated to abnormalities in immune system, neurotransmitters and anatomical changes. Anatomical abnormalities have been identified in schizophrenics through neuroimaging techniques in which decreased brain volume, changes in hippocampus and larger ventricles are the main anatomical abnormalities (Mattai, Hosanagar, Weisinger, Greenstein, Stidd &

6

Clasen, 2010). Recent studies indicate that changes in prefrontal lobes among people with schizophrenia are responsible for increased severity of the main symptoms (McIntosh, Owens, Moorhead, Whalley, Stanfield & Hall, 2011). On the other hand, abnormalities in the dopaminergic system have been found to be responsible for the pathophysiology of schizophrenia. For instance, neurotransmitter substances, especially N -methyl-D-aspartate (NMDA) and its antagonists such as ketamine and phencyclidine are linked to the development of schizophrenic negative symptoms (Cioffi, 2013). Moreover, abnormalities in the immune system, especially its overactivation by stress or prenatal infection, play key roles in the pathophysiology of schizophrenia. Drexhage et al. (2011) report that schizophrenics show disturbed immune function with an active kynurenine pathway which is responsible for inflammation responses.

Treatment of Schizophrenia

In practice, the treatment of schizophrenia involves the use of antipsychotic medications and psychosocial interventions.

Antipsychotic Medication

Antipsychotics have become the mainstay of schizophrenia treatment, and they are meant to address the symptoms of the disorder. For instance, the positive symptoms of schizophrenia can be treated with medications such as olanzapine, aripiprazole, quetiapine, Risperidone, and ziprasidone. Other effective medications for treating positive symptoms include iloperidone, lurasidone, asenapine, and paliperidone. However, it is worth noting that these medications may cause side effects. Some the common side effects include dizziness, sleepiness, elevated blood sugar and lipids, weight gain, and increased appetite (Lehman et al., 2010).

In order to treat schizophrenia-related depression, antidepressant medications are used. Some of these medications include fluoxetine, escitalopram, paroxetine, sertraline, bupropion, duloxetine, citalopram, and venlafaxine (Lehman et al., 2010).

Psychosocial Interventions

Psychosocial interventions are considered essential in the management of schizophrenia. Some of the main interventions include family psycho-education, assertive community treatment (ACT), substance abuse treatment, social skills training, supported employment, and cognitive behavioral therapy (CBT) (Lehman et al., 2010).

CBT is aimed at improving the patient's social interactions through addressing the negative symptoms such as social withdrawal and disturbed attention. As such, this therapy acts as a reality-based intervention. Similarly, social skills training enables patients to cope with the social problems associated with schizophrenia, especially improving relationships with other people, including family members and healthcare personnel. On the other hand, assertive community treatment involves improving the patient's interactions within the community settings through the use of a treatment team, whereas family psycho-education involves teaching family members the key aspects of the disorder, in order to enhance treatment. When family psycho-education intervention is carried out effectively, chances of schizophrenia's relapse have been found to be very minimal. Psycho-education has also been found to reduce schizophrenia symptoms and rehospityalization (Xia, Merinder & Belgamwar, 2011).

Prognosis

From a clinical perspective, guarding of prognosis of schizophrenia is necessary because full recovery is rare. Ordinarily, individuals with early schizophrenia onset, severe cognitive symptoms, abnormalities in brain structure, and family history of the illness experience poor prognosis. On the other hand, it is reported that people living in middle and low-income countries experience better prognosis (Haro, Novick & Bertsch, 2011).

In addition, poor access to medical care among schizophrenics contributes to the severity of the illness owing to the loss of disease control approaches. As a result, patients are prone to incarceration and homelessness due to poverty. It is also reported that schizophrenics have an increased mortality due to factors such as lack of exercise, poor nutrition and cigarette smoking. Moreover, suicide is responsible for mortality with lifetime risk of suicide among schizophrenics estimated to be 5% (Hoang, Stewart & Goldacre, 2011).

Current Research Directions

Currently, extensive research is ongoing to improve understanding and treatment of schizophrenia. For instance, new agents for treating schizophrenia are on clinical trials. One of such agents is minocycline which has been found to have beneficial effects in treatment of the disorder (Dean, Data-Franco, Giorlando & Berk, 2012). Another research direction related to schizophrenia is the use of Nidotherapy which focuses on improving the functioning of schizophrenics.

Conclusion

Conclusively, schizophrenia emerges as one of the mental health disorders that pose immense challenges to healthcare personnel, individuals and families. This illness affects all people, but its onset is rare during early childhood.

Clinical studies indicate that the causes of schizophrenia are associated with environmental and genetic factors. In addition, abnormalities in the brain chemistry and structure are also responsible for the occurrence of the disorder. The disease's onset involves an early phase of warning signs that signal impairment in an individual's cognitive functioning. However, the main symptoms include disorganized speech or behavior, hallucinations and delusions.

Diagnosis is based on the main symptoms, whereas its treatment focuses on addressing the symptoms. Treatment combines antipsychotic medications with psychosocial interventions. However, it is worth noting that new diagnostic and treatment approaches are emerging from scientific inquiry related to schizophrenia.

References

American Psychiatric Association (2000). *Diagnostic and statistical manual of mental disorders (DSM-IV-TR). 4th ed.* Washington, DC: American Psychiatric Press.

Cascio, M., Cella, M., Preti, A., Meneghelli, A., & Cocchi, A. (2012). Gender and duration of untreated psychosis: a systematic review and meta-analysis. *Early Intervention In Psychiatry (Review)*, 6(2), 115–27. doi:10.1111/j.1751-7893.2012.00351.x

Cioffi, C. L. (2013). Modulation of NMDA receptor function as a treatment for schizophrenia. *Bioorg Med Chem Lett.*, 23(18), 5034-5044.

Dean, O. M., Data-Franco, J., Giorlando, F., & Berk, M. (2012). Minocycline: therapeutic potential in psychiatry. *CNS Drugs*, 26(5), 391–401. doi: 10.2165/11632000-000000000-00000

Drexhage, R. C., Weigelt, K., van Beveren, N., Cohen, D., Versnel, M. A., & Nolen, W. (2011). Immune and neuroimmune alterations in mood disorders and schizophrenia. *Int Rev Neurobiol.*, 101, 169-201.

Haro, J. M., Novick, D., & Bertsch, J. (2011). Cross-national clinical and functional remission rates: Worldwide Schizophrenia Outpatient Health Outcomes (W-SOHO) study. *Br J Psychiatry*, 199, 194-201.

Hoang, U., Stewart, R., Goldacre, M. J. (2011). Mortality after hospital discharge for people with schizophrenia or bipolar disorder: retrospective study of linked English hospital episode statistics, 1999-2006. *BMJ, 343,* d5422.

Kumra, S., Shaw, M., Merka, P., Nakayama, E., & Augustin, R. (2001). Childhood-onset schizophrenia: research update. *Canadian Journal of Psychiatry*, 46(10), 923–30.

Lehman, A., Lieberman, J., Dixon, L., McGlashan, T., Miller, A., Perkins, D., & Kreyenbuhl, J. (2010). *Practice guideline for the treatment of patients with schizophrenia 2nd edn.* Washington, DC: American Psychiatric Press.

Lozano, R., Naghavi, M., & Foreman, K. (2012). Global and regional mortality from 235 causes of death for 20 age groups in 1990 and 2010: a systematic analysis for the Global Burden of Disease Study 2010, *Lancet*, 380(9859), 2095–128. doi:10.1016/S0140-6736(12)61728-0

Mattai, A., Hosanagar, A., Weisinger, B., Greenstein, D., Stidd, R., & Clasen. L. (2011). Hippocampal volume development in healthy siblings of childhood-onset schizophrenia patients. *Am J Psychiatry*, 168(4), 427-35.

McIntosh, A. M., Owens, D., Moorhead, W., Whalley, H., Stanfield, A., & Hall, J. (2011). Longitudinal volume reductions in people at high genetic risk of schizophrenia as they develop psychosis. *Biol Psychiatry*, 69(10), 953-8.

Picchioni, M., & Murray, R. M. (2007). Schizophrenia. *BMJ, 335,* (7610), 91–5. doi:10.1136/bmj.39227.616447.

Van Os, J., & Kapur, S. (2009). Schizophrenia. *Lancet*, 374(9690), 635–45. doi:10.1016/S0140-6736(09)60995-8

Wright, C., Rabe-Hesketh, S., & Woodruff, W. (2000). Meta-analysis of regional brain volumes in schizophrenia. *Am J Psychiatry*, 157(1), 16-25.

Xia, J., Merinder, L., & Belgamwar, M. (2011). Psychoeducation for schizophrenia. *Cochrane Database Syst Rev.*, 15(6), CD002831.

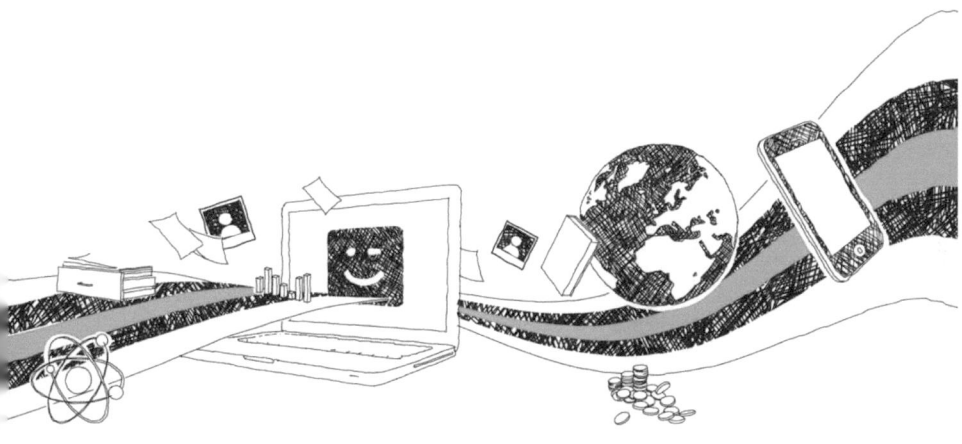
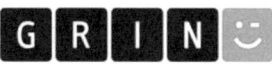